D0717402

OFFICE

Relaxation

Simple Meditations and Yoga Stretches for the Workplace

by Darrin Zeer
illustrations by Michael Klein and Frank Montagna

Copyright © 2001, 2002 by **Darrin Zeer.**
Illustrations copyright © 2001 by **Michael Klein** (pages 1–51),
© 2002 by **Frank Montagna** (pages 52–96).
All rights reserved.
No part of this book may be reproduced in any form without
written permission from the publisher.

Manufactured in China.

Produced exclusively for **Marks and Spencer p.l.c.**
by **Chronicle Books LLC,** San Francisco, California.

British Library Catalogue-in-Publication Data.
A catalogue record for this book is available from the British Library.

THIS BOOK IS DEDICATED TO ALL OF YOU.

May it inspire you to

take good care of yourself

at the office and throughout the day.

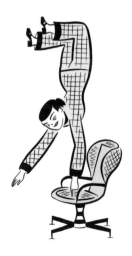

C ntents

QUick *HELP guide*

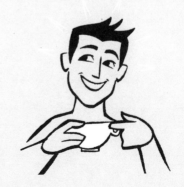

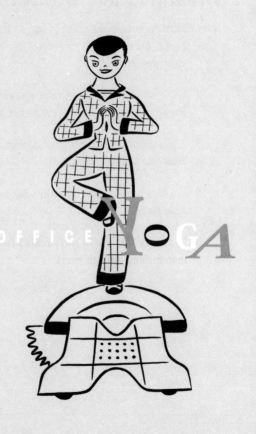

OFFICE Y·O·GA

Five Essential Tips for Breathing and Stretching

1. Most important: When stretching, do not hold your breath. Breathe deeply and slowly, in rhythm with your movements.

2. While stretching, focus on relaxing your entire body. Pay attention to the areas that remain tense.

3. If you want to go deeper into a stretch, breathe and relax into it. Don't force it.

4. If a stretch hurts, don't do it. In other words: "If pain, no gain."

5. In a hurry? Do one or two stretches fully rather than rushing through many.

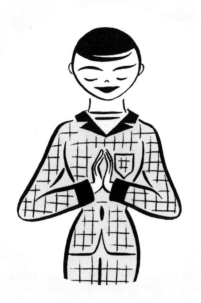

Gentle Sun Salutations

1.

This gentle series of yoga postures helps wake up the entire body. Take the first round slow and easy; if you become dizzy, lie flat on your back and rest. As you become more adept at the postures, your breath should fall into a rhythm like the waves of the ocean.

First, place your hands in a prayer position and inhale deeply. Reach your hands up high and stretch, arching slightly back. Exhaling, sweep your outstretching arms forward and down till you are bent over, touching the floor if you can; relax your head and neck and take a few breaths. Squat down, place your hands flat on the ground, take a big step back with your left foot, and stretch, arching up with your back. Step back with your right foot and rest both knees on the ground, making a table with your body; first stretch your head up and curve your lower back down, then drop your head down and arch your back up. Repeat once and breathe in rhythm as you do.

With your hands and the soles of your feet on the ground, lift your buttocks toward the sky, keeping your arms and legs straight and your heels down; stay as long as comfortable. Drop down onto your hands and knees,

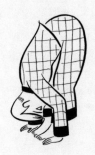

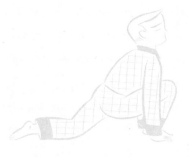

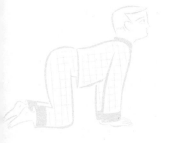

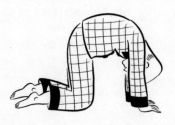

6.

sit on your calves, and lower your upper body to the ground with your arms outstretched on the floor. Relax for a few breaths. Raise back up on your hands and knees and bring your left foot forward, so it's underneath you, with your right leg stretched back. Arch your back upward and breathe. Bring your right foot forward, straighten your legs with your upper body hanging down, and slowly walk your hands up your legs into a standing position. Raise your arms toward the sky and stretch back slightly, tightening your buttocks. Exhale as you return your hands to the beginning prayer position, then relax.

Rest for a few moments, breathing deeply and rhythmically, then repeat as many times as you want or as time permits.

7.

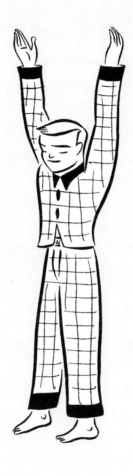

8

Red Light Rejuvenation

This also works on planes and trains.

Sit back, relax, and gently roll your head in circles.

Shrug your shoulders up and down, breathing in rhythm as you do.

Become one with the traffic flow.

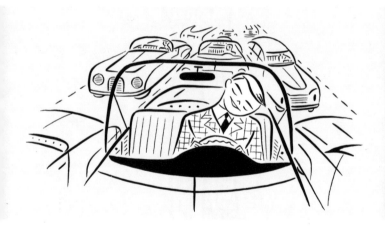

Antidote for Road Rage

Stop-and-go traffic making you nuts? Loosen up your windpipes and sing your favorite song. Imitate an opera singer and come from your belly with the sound.

"Better late than never."

—*Titus Livius*

Office Yoga Posture

Want to ease your back pain and improve and energize
your mood at the same time? Good posture is the best
start. Throughout the day and when preparing for your
Office Yoga stretches, take a moment to align your
body properly.

> **Most important is to sit on your sit bones; to
> find these sharp bones, place your hands under
> your buttocks and rock forward and back.**
>
> **Notice how, when you rise forward, your body
> aligns on top of your sit bones; immediately
> your back straightens, your chest expands, and
> your shoulders, neck, and head rise and align.**
>
> **Now sit back on your tailbone—everything
> slumps and drops, including your mood!**
>
> **Rise forward again. Feel your spine lift into a
> straight line all the way up to your head.**
>
> **Let your shoulders relax, soften your jaw, lower
> your chin, and take a few deep calm breaths.**

Can you feel the difference? This simple shift in posture improves not only your physical well-being but
your confidence and sense of self.

Keyboard Calisthenics

Do stretches with your hands and wrists as often as possible. Improvise–be creative!

With hands in a prayer position, move in all directions and stretch.

Squeeze fists tight.

Stretch fingers wide.

Interlace fingers and rotate hands.

Invent stretches that feel good.

Make it a habit: Constantly stretch your hands and wrists.

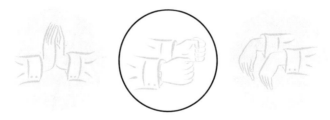

"Common sense is not so common."

–Voltaire

Neck Rolls

Drop your head to one side.

Roll it around in a wide circle; switch directions.

Slowly find the tight spots.

Hold and breathe, letting your breath release the tightness.

Extra stretch: Place a hand on your head and gently pull to the side.

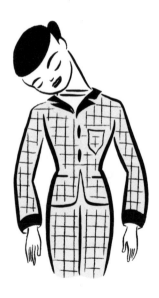

Arm Pulls

Place left arm behind your back.

Grab your wrist with your right hand.

Drop your head to the right side.

Roll head slightly and explore any tightness.

Stretch and breathe.

Repeat with other arm.

Bend left arm above and behind your head.

Grab your elbow with your right hand and stretch up.

Breathe and let shoulders relax.

Repeat with other arm.

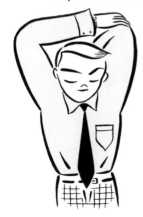

Kick Back Log-on Pose

Interlace your fingers behind your head.

Relax your elbows and shoulders.

Smile, breathe, and stretch your elbows back.

Let the tightness release slowly.

Repeat throughout the day.

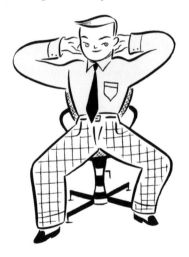

"Let the beauty of what you love be what you do."

−Rumi

Human Basketball Net

Raise your arms straight above your head.

Interlace your fingers.

Alternate palms downward and upward.

Stretch and breathe.

Stretch your arms out in front and relax your shoulders.

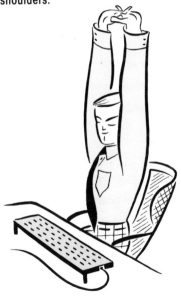

Reaching Hands

First Stretch:

> Hold your arms out to the side.
>
> Stretch with your fingertips to the opposite walls.
>
> Breathe and relax.

Second Stretch:

> Arms outstretched, shoulders relaxed, palms down.
>
> Tilt hands upward and stretch forearms.
>
> Hold as long as comfortable.
>
> Stretch hands down, breathe, and hold.

Third Stretch:

> Arms outstretched.
>
> Slowly tilt sideways like a windmill.
>
> Reach for the floor and ceiling.
>
> Gently stretch the mid-area.

"Learning is movement from moment to moment."

−Krishnamurti

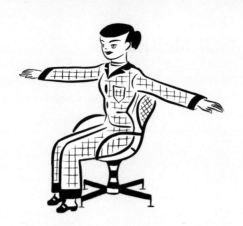

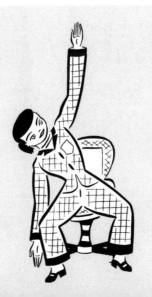

E-mail Meditation

While you are reading your e-mail, remember to breathe slowly and focus your attention on your breath. Make the out-breath two times longer than the in-breath. This will immediately calm you.

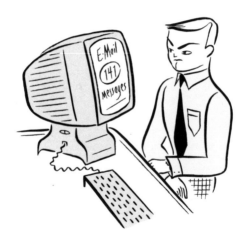

"Kind words can be short and easy to speak, but their echoes are truly endless."

—Mother Teresa

Open Chest Stretch

Sit near the edge of the chair.

Hold the sides of the seat.

Gently stretch up and forward.

Open your chest and tilt your head back.

Relax and breathe into the stretch.

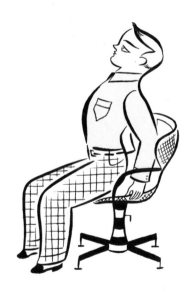

Circling Torso

Sit forward with your feet flat on the ground, hands on hips (if you can), and relax your shoulders. Begin to rotate your torso in circles. Explore with your whole body, relax, and breathe.

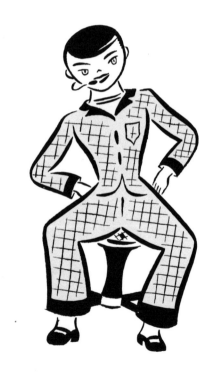

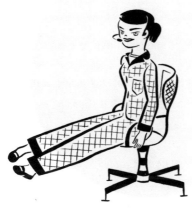

Feet and Ankles

While you talk on the phone, stretch your legs out and
rotate your ankles and feet. Notice your attention
increase as you stretch.

Balance Tree Pose

Try this just before a big meeting or call.

- Remove shoes and stand next to a table or chair for balance.

- Raise right foot up against the inside of thigh.

- Place right hand on foot if it slides down.

- If you feel steady, place hands by chest in prayer position.

- Feel the standing foot rooted into the ground.

- Relax and breathe.

- Stand straight and balanced.

- Switch legs slowly.

"Do it big, do it right, and do it with style."

—Fred Astaire

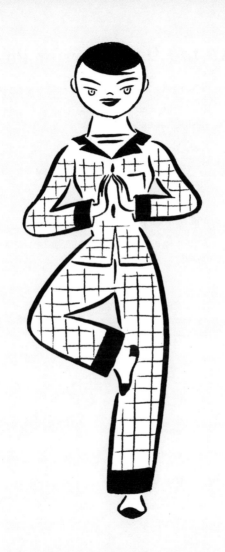

Close the Deal Warrior Pose

Raise your arms to the side with fingers pointed.

Take a big step to the side, with your right foot turned out and knee bent.

Keep your left foot planted, your leg straight.

Your upper body should be straight and strong, shoulders relaxed.

Don't hold your breath! Relax into the stretch and then gently release.

Return to a standing position, switch sides, and repeat.

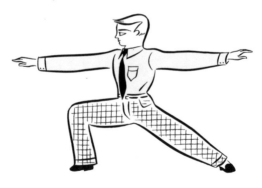

"Make haste slowly."

—Zen master

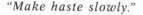

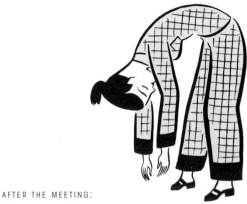

Ragdoll Pose

Let it all out with this re-energizing stretch.

> Take a deep breath.
>
> Arms straight up and stretch.
>
> Exhale, bend knees, and drop hands to ground.
>
> Relax your head and shoulders and take deep full-body breaths.
>
> Let everything sag toward the ground while still bent over.
>
> Return to standing position by slowly walking hands up legs.

Cobra Pose

Change into sweats at lunch and keep your back
healthy with this series of stretches.

Beginner's Cobra

Lie on your stomach, your forearms on the
ground.

Keep your elbows beneath your shoulders,
slightly supporting your raised upper body.

Keep your hips on the ground and your buttocks
tight to support your lower back.

Gently lift your head and chest.

Breathe and stretch, letting the tight areas
release.

Hold and breathe.

When ready, gently lower yourself to the ground.
Repeat.

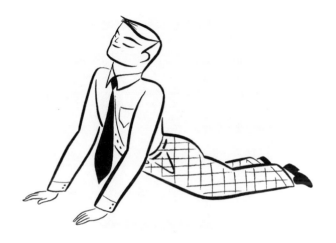

Full Cobra

Practice this stretch if the Beginner's Cobra is easy, but skip if you have lower back problems.

> Lie on stomach, hands under shoulders, palms down, elbows in.
>
> Lift your head and chest by slowly contracting your lower back muscles.
>
> Use your arm strength for support.
>
> Breathe deeply and relax.

Cat Pose

Get on your hands and knees to begin each Cat Pose.

Cat Cow

> Raise your head up and arch your lower back down.
>
> Exhale as you drop your head and arch your lower back up.
>
> Move slowly, stretch deeply.
>
> Repeat.

Cat Stretch

> Gently lower your body onto your calves with your arms stretched out.
>
> Relax your head and neck.
>
> Breathe and rest. Feel your lower back release.

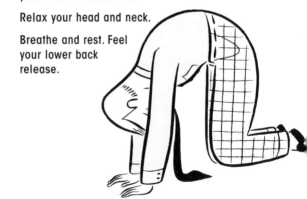

Belly and *Hips*

Lie on your back to begin each of the following
Healthy Back Stretches.

Half Sit-Ups

Bend legs and cross arms over chest.

Breathe deep and slowly sit halfway up.

Pause. Feel your belly tighten.

Breathe, release, rest, and repeat.

Hip Raises

Bend legs, arms at your side and palms down.

Gently raise your hips and hold.

Breathe, release, and repeat.

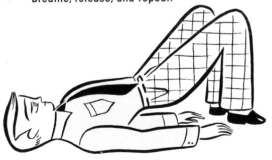

Knees Up

Sometimes the most powerful stretches are the easiest ones.

> Interlace fingers or arms around bent knees.
>
> Gently stretch your knees to chest, keeping your hips on the floor.
>
> Hold the stretch. Breathe into your lower back.
>
> Relax your body, and rest in the pose.

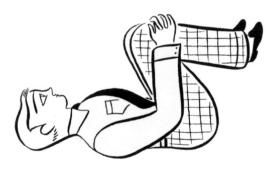

"Work is love made visible."

–Kahlil Gibran

Child's Posture

This is a gentle, relaxing stretch for your lower back.

Sit on calves and lay upper body on legs.

Place arms at your side.

Turn face to one side or lay forehead on ground.

Let your body relax and breathe.

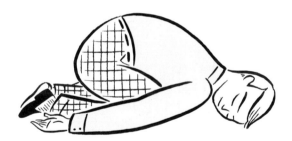

Crowded Elevator *Stretch*

Place hand on a wall for balance.

Standing on your left foot, cross right foot over left leg just above the ground.

Feel the sole of your left foot rooted into the floor, lengthen your body.

Relax and breathe, then switch legs.

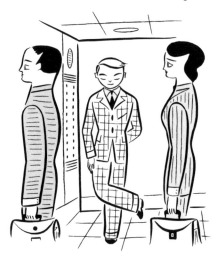

"To be uncertain is uncomfortable, but to be certain is ridiculous."

—Chinese proverb

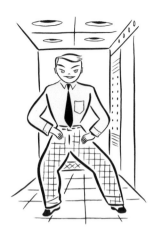

Empty Elevator *Stretches*

Place your right hand on a wall.

Stand up straight and bend your left leg back.

With your left hand, hold your toes and pull your foot to your buttocks.

Breathe, hold, release, and switch sides.

Place your hands on your hips.

With your legs apart, bend both knees slightly.

Make wide circles with your hips.

Reverse directions and breathe.

Photocopier Stretch

Place your hands on the edge of the copier.

Stand back with feet apart.

Drop your head and chest.

Breathe and relax your shoulders.

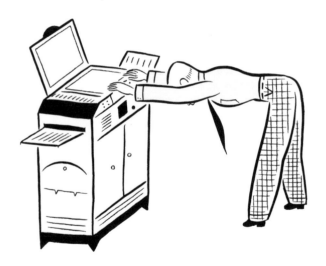

Late Client *Stretch*

Place both hands on the doorjambs at shoulder height, feet hip-width apart.

Gently let your body stretch forward.

Relax your head and breathe.

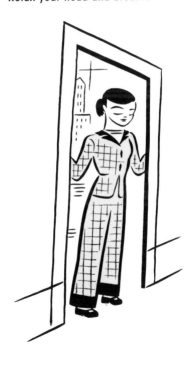

Energize Anytime

Shake your hands and arms.

Shake each leg and foot, one at a time.

Swing your arms in wide circles—up and around and from side to side.

Switch directions.

Wiggle your whole body till it feels loose.

Raise both arms above your head.

Take left wrist with your right hand and gently stretch to the right.

Breathe into the stretch.

Keep your body straight and strong.

Switch sides and repeat.

"No act of kindness, no matter how small, is ever wasted."

– Aesop

Hands Behind *Back*

Interlace your fingers behind your back.

Gently bend forward.

Stretch your hands and arms up and back.

Breathe into the stretch.

Gently release arms.

With fists, tap lower back and legs.

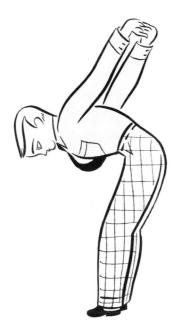

On-the-Run *Stretch*

Lift your right foot onto a solid desk or table.

Turn your standing foot to the side for balance.

Stretch over your leg, placing your hands on your leg or on the table.

Relax your head. Breathe into the stretch.

Flex your foot, breathe.

Relax your foot, breathe.

Switch legs and repeat.

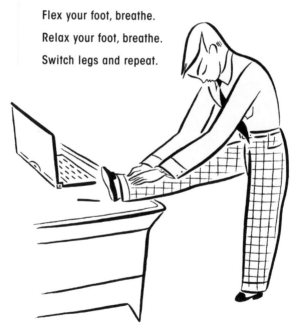

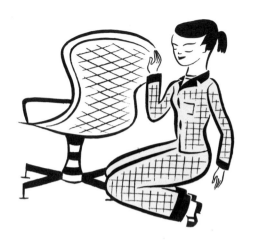

Power Leg Bends

Place your hand on a solid chair to steady yourself.

Keeping your back straight, bend your knees, lower body slowly, and then raise up.

Do this several times slowly, breathing in rhythm.

Try this with your feet down or heels up.

"The moment we want to be something we are no longer free."

–Krishnamurti

Let It Go, Let It Out

When you're done for the day, release all your tension.

> While sitting, reach your hands toward the sky.
>
> Breathe in deeply and relax completely on the exhale.
>
> Drop your arms and upper body toward the ground like a rag doll.

Make sure you're alone before trying this Lion Pose!

> While at your desk, take a deep breath and roar as loud as you can. Come from your belly with the sound, and open your mouth as wide as you can.

"He who knows others is wise;
He who knows himself is enlightened."

—Lao-tzu

Breathing Meditation

Place one hand on your belly.

Breathe slow and deep.

Feel your hand rise and fall.

Let your shoulders drop.

Feel your body relax and renew.

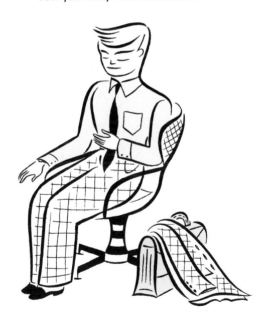

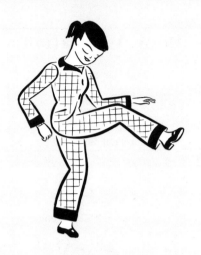

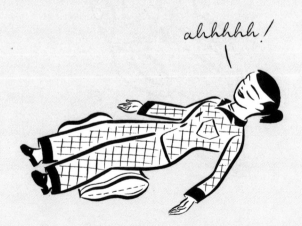

ahhhhh!

Getting Home *Release*

Twist and Shout

Put on your favorite music, and for two to five minutes, simply let your hair down. Free-flow dance and stretch. Focus on letting go of your day and relaxing.

Rest and Relax

For two to five minutes, lie down on your back and let your thoughts go. Get comfortable, perhaps placing a pillow under your knees. Take easy breaths. Imagine your body sinking into the ground. Relax the tight spots, calm the mind, feel peace.

OFFICE *Spa*

the FIVE *golden RULES*
of the OFFICE *spa*

I
    I will breathe deeply and slowly,
                  relaxing my body.

2
    I will keep things simple,
                  moving forward one step at a time.

3
    I will focus on each step calmly.

4
    I will not stress out about
                  the little things.

5
    I will treat myself to an *Office Spa*
                  break whenever the need arises.

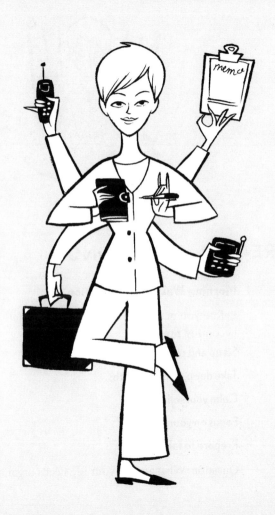

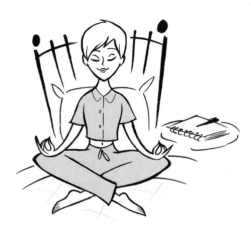

PRE-work *PAMPERING*

Morning Wake-up Meditation

Before you get out of bed, spend ten minutes becoming present.

1 Sit up and relax your body.

2 Take deep, gentle breaths.

3 Calm yourself.

4 Focus on your day.

5 Prepare to take action.

Question: What area of your life needs organizing?

CAR Comfort

Why not turn your vehicle into a sanctuary? Make an altar by placing a flower or your favorite picture on your dashboard. Create scents and sounds that are personal and peaceful. Challenge yourself to remain calm and enjoy the moment as you move through rush-hour traffic. Driving is a meditation on staying sharp and alert to your surroundings. Keep a small carry bag handy with a nice change of clothes and a toiletry kit in it. Relaxation is being prepared for the unexpected. Your car is also a great place to escape to during the day when you need peace, quiet, and privacy.

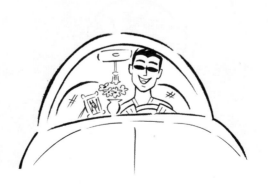

MORNING blues

Need a quick pick-me-up? Stimulate your senses with aromatherapy. The oldest form of medicine known to human-kind, aromatherapy promotes health and well-being through the use of essential oils, the most concentrated essence of a plant. Ylang-ylang essential oil has a soft fragrance that helps calm anxiety. You can purchase a small vial at a health-food store or beauty shop. Store it in a desk drawer, and when you arrive at work in the morning, open the bottle and take a whiff.

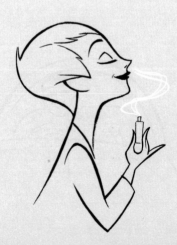

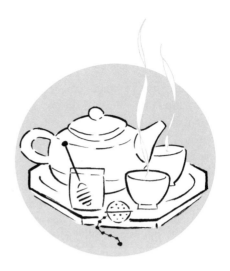

HERbal *TEA ceremony*

Are you ready to go beyond the tea bag? Create a "tea corner" on your desk with a nice Japanese or English teapot, some teacups, honey, and a selection of teas.

When you are ready for a break with a co-worker or client, share some tea. Get out a tea ball or strainer to hold the herbs. Add 2 tablespoons of herbs for each cup and place inside the teapot. Pour hot water into the pot, cover, and let steep for a few minutes.

Pour the tea into the cups and sweeten if desired. Peace can come from simple activities.

say "CHI"

In many parts of Asia it is believed that good health is maintained by a flow of energy called *chi*. By pressing particular points on the face you can stimulate *chi*, relieve tension, and bring a glow to your cheeks. Let your fingers do the walking.

1   With the pointer finger of each hand, find a spot on each side of your face and press gently but firmly for a few moments. Do not rub or scrub. Continue by pressing different spots around your face.

2   With your fingertips, rhythmically tap all over your face like raindrops.

3   To stimulate circulation, gently pound your cheeks and forehead with loose fists.

4   End the treatment by gently placing your hands over your face to soothe.

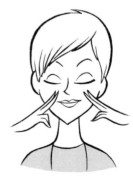

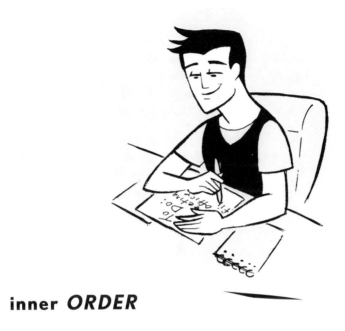

inner *ORDER*

Your workweek will go much more smoothly if you take
some time in the morning to write your anxieties away.
Appointments, to-do lists, deadlines—get these out
of your head and onto paper and you'll feel the stress fade
away. Check items off throughout the day and see how
much you accomplish.

STAY *on* the BALL

Work out while you're working! Swiss balls are large, inflated rubber balls that are available at any back-care store. Sitting atop the ball helps your posture by forcing you to constantly shift to maintain your balance. For maximum benefits, use the Swiss ball for your desk chair.

Feeling frustrated? Bounce!

1 Sit comfortably on the ball with your back straight. Imagine a string is attached to the top of your head, pulling your head straight up toward the ceiling.

2 Bend your knees and spread your feet wide until you find your balance.

3 Bounce slowly and breathe.

You'll be surprised at the workout you can get!

 Confine yourself to the present.

—Marcus Aurelius

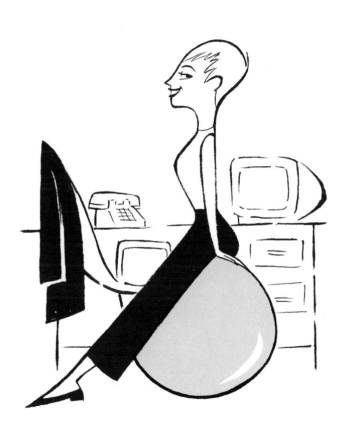

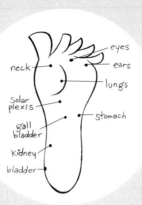

- eyes
- ears
- neck
- lungs
- Solar plexis
- stomach
- gall bladder
- kidney
- bladder

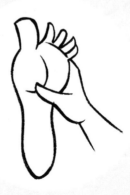

relaxing REFLEXology

Reflexology is the art of applying pressure to specific points on the feet to assist circulation and ease aches and pains in the body. The quick reflexology routine given below is easy to do anytime. Since there are thousands of nerve endings on the feet, it's hard to "miss the point."

1. Remove your shoes.

2. Cross one leg over the other, resting your ankle comfortably just above your knee.

3. Relax as you begin to knead your foot, using the strength of your thumbs to apply pressure to the spots given in the diagram.

4. Take it easy; don't hurt yourself. To apply more pressure, use your knuckles.

5. When you find a sensitive spot, hold the pressure and take deep, gentle breaths.

6. Work in a circular motion over your entire foot.

7. To finish, knead in larger circles, moving above your ankles to your calves.

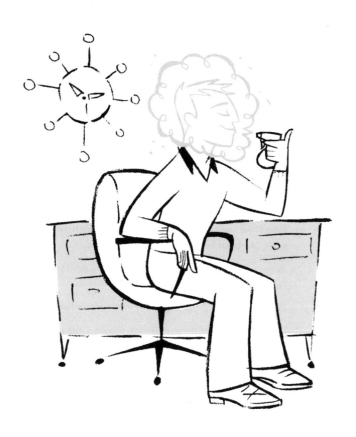

Meeting *MIST*

Let lavender set the mood! The scent of lavender alleviates stress-related symptoms such as headaches, insomnia, anxiety, and fatigue.

1. Fill a clean spray bottle with 6–8 tablespoons of cool water.

2. Add 2–4 drops of lavender essential oil and shake.

3. With your eyes closed, mist your face.

4. Take a nice deep breath.

5. Organize your thoughts and spend a moment focusing on your agenda.

6. Keep the bottle tightly closed and treat yourself and your desk area to a spritz throughout the day.

Tension is who you think you should be.
Relaxation is who you are. —Chinese Proverb

KEYboard *recovery*

To avoid computer strain and keep your hands in mint con-
dition, take a break after every 15 minutes of typing. Make
the most of your breaks by giving yourself a helping hand.
Keep your favorite moisturizer at your desk and give yourself a soothing hand massage. Working certain pressure
points can help relieve work stress.

1 Spread moisturizer thickly onto your hands.

2 Interlace your fingers and using your thumb,
massage the palm of your other hand.

3 For deeper treatment, search out sore spots, press
with the thumb, and hold for 10 seconds.

4 Once you've found all the sore spots, switch hands.

5 Remember to breathe deeply into your belly and
relax your shoulders while massaging.

6 To complete, interlace your fingers and squeeze and
massage both hands at once.

7 Notice the fast tension relief!

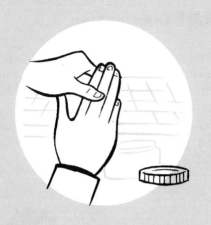

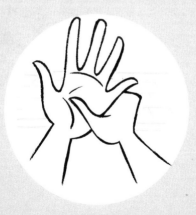

INSTANT *inspiration*

Need a refreshing inspiration for your next project?
Eucalyptus essential oil will help clear your thoughts. Dab
a few drops on a piece of paper and breathe in the aroma.
If you feel congested or sense a cold coming on, put 4
drops of eucalyptus in a cup of hot water. (For increased
effectiveness, place a towel over your head and breathe in
the steam.) The strong scent will revive you.

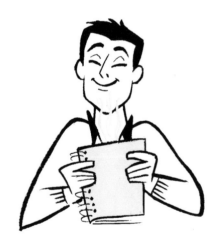

 Worry often gives a small thing a big shadow.

—Swedish Proverb

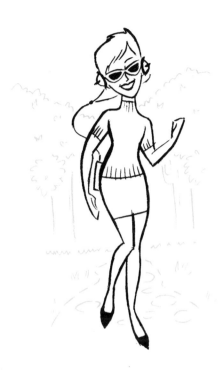

Take a WALK on the *WILD SIDE*

Getting too intimate with your desk? Becoming codependent with your computer? Time to make a run for it! For a heavy dose of nature, take yourself to the local park. Just a few minutes in a green space will put things into perspective.

If the SHOE *FITS*, wear *it!*

In an average day, a person will take more than 7,000 steps. In an average lifetime, a person will walk more than 100,000 miles. The message: Be good to your feet and they'll serve you well for miles to come. Here are a couple of tips:

1. Keep a pair of running shoes at your desk for unexpected errands. If your shoes are comfortable, you'll be inspired to walk farther.

2. For those of you burning the midnight oil, keep a pair of cozy slippers at your desk. When the office starts to quiet down, take off your shoes and put on your fuzzy slippers. Your feet will thank you.

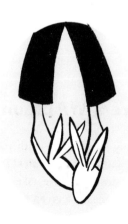

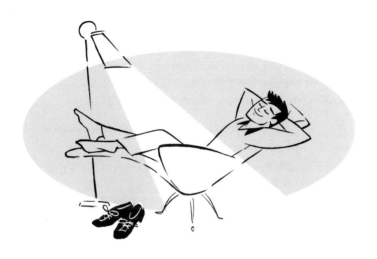

POST-meeting *POWER NAP*

Research shows that when your energy wanes and your
creativity is stifled, an afternoon nap can be just the cure.
Some companies even have nap rooms with lounge chairs
and peaceful music. Others have a comfortable couch or
chair in the lunchroom. Seek out a quiet nook, maybe even
a bench outside in the sun. Set your watch alarm and let
yourself drift off. Even five minutes can make a difference.

Acu*PRESSURE* *in the* AFTERnoon

Taking your shoes off when walking around the office or when sitting at your desk can be very rejuvenating and helpful for sore feet. For extra relief for backaches and headaches, try this easy under-the-desk technique.

1 Place a golf ball or rolling pin on the floor under your feet.

2 While sitting, roll the sole of each foot firmly over the ball or rolling pin.

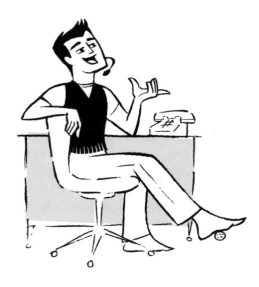

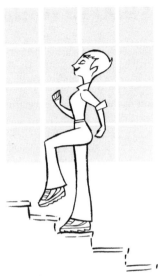

WALK *your* *WORRIES* away

Something troubling you? A deadline? Too many to-do's? A co-worker? Refresh yourself and get some exercise, too, by taking a brisk walk. Put on your walking shoes and try climbing some stairs. Bring your knees up high for an extra challenge. Walk it off. Or, for a gentler workout, take a tour around the office. Walk slowly and step out of your troubles by focusing on each step. Feel the entire sole of each foot as it touches the ground. By the end of your walk, your troubles will have gone. Move on to the next task with enthusiasm!

SHIATSU tension **TAMER**

Shiatsu is a Japanese finger pressure massage. It encourages the flow of energy in the body. This self-treatment is very energizing and stress relieving. It doesn't require massage oil and can easily be performed over clothing. Try it on your arms, legs, or wherever you feel a muscle ache.

1   Get comfortable in your seat.

2   Begin to relax your body, muscle by muscle.

3   Press your thumb or fingertips into any area where muscles are tight.

4   Apply firm pressure for five seconds, then move to another spot.

5   Take a deep breath and focus on relaxing your body as you apply the pressure.

Don't be surprised if you feel the benefits immediately!

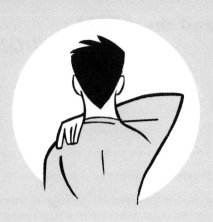

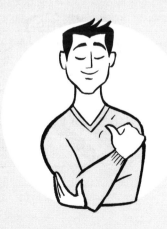

ZEN and the *ART of organizaTION*

A clean desk makes for a clear mind. Create order in a calm, meditative way.

    1 Pay attention to the busyness of your mind.

    2 What judgments or frustrations do you carry?

    3 Breathe in rhythm to your movements.

    4 Enjoy the challenge of bringing your space into perfect order. Every item has its proper place.

When finished, your mind will feel open and light.

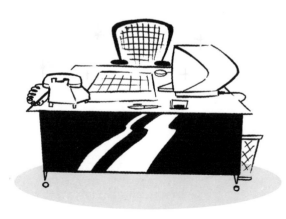

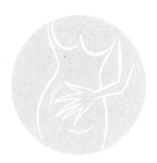

HARA power

When it comes to massage, the abdominal area rarely gets any attention. Stomach massage can provide relief for indigestion, tension, and menstrual cramps. In Japan the entire stomach area is referred to as the *hara,* and it is considered to be the energy center for the entire body. To massage yourself:

Place the palm of your hand near your navel.

Make gentle circles around your navel in a clockwise motion.

Try pressing with your fingertips as you continue to slowly circle.

If you find a sore spot, stop and hold the pressure for a moment, and breathe deeply into your belly.

At the end of the session hold your hand still over your navel for a few moments.

Take deep breaths, and let your shoulders relax.

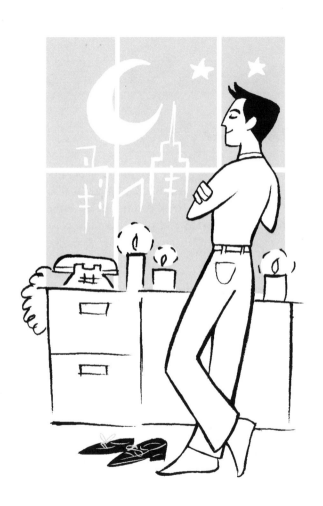

BURNING the *MIDNIGHT* OIL
spa kit

Keep these supplies handy for those unavoidable late nights.

- ✳ Fuzzy slippers
- ✳ Candles
- ✳ Sparkling water
- ✳ To-go menus from your favorite restaurants
- ✳ Energy bars
- ✳ Getting sleepy? Do a sound check in the office and turn up the tunes!

Remember when you were at your best?
Now be there again! —Author unknown

ELEVate *your MIND*

The elevator is one area with no distractions. Take a ride for some time out.

1 Position yourself at the rear of the elevator.

2 Stand comfortably with your knees slightly bent.

3 Watch the numbers rise or fall in unison with your breath.

4 When your floor arrives you will be calm and centered.

You can't do it right, you can't get it wrong.
You can only let go. —The Lady

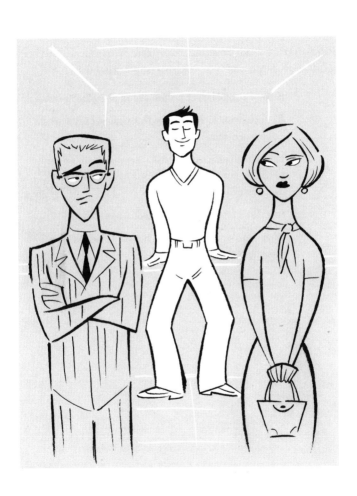

CHAMOMILE *compress*

Still suffering from computer eyestrain? Chamomile reduces swelling and is a very relaxing herbal drink.

1. Brew a cup of hot chamomile tea using two tea bags.

2. Remove the tea bags from the cup and set aside to cool on a plate.

3. When the tea bags are still warm but cool enough to touch, lean back, close your eyes, and gently place one bag onto each eyelid.

4. Rest for a few minutes with your eyes closed.

5. When the eye compresses have cooled, remove them and enjoy your tea.

All comes at the proper time to him who knows how to wait. —Saint Vincent de Paul

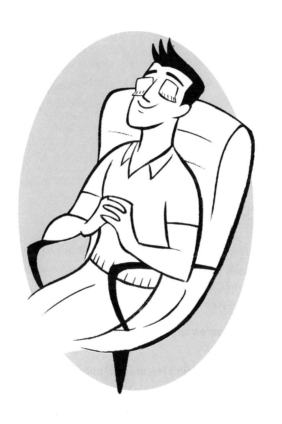

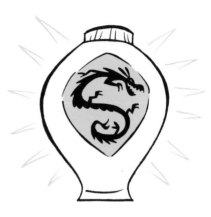

GINSENG *zing*

Is your aching body keeping you pinned to your seat?
For centuries ginseng has been recognized for its energizing properties. It provides a great boost when you need to bench-press your tired body out of your chair.

1 Prepare a hot cup of ginseng tea (available at most stores).

2 Try putting in a few drops of pure ginseng extract for an extra kick.

3 Add some honey or maple syrup.

4 Take a deep breath, and wait for the power surge.

EYE *energizer*

Tired eyes are a common side effect of computer use. Often, people forget to blink when staring at a computer screen.

To alleviate eyestrain and stress:

1. Refocus every ten minutes by looking out the window or around the office.
2. Roll your eyes in a circles, making sure to roll in both directions.
3. Once an hour close your eyes and let your face relax.

For soothing relief:

1. Rub your palms together quickly to warm them.
2. Place your palms gently over your closed eyes.
3. Hold them over your eyes until the heat dissipates.
4. Take a relaxing breath.

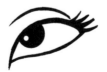

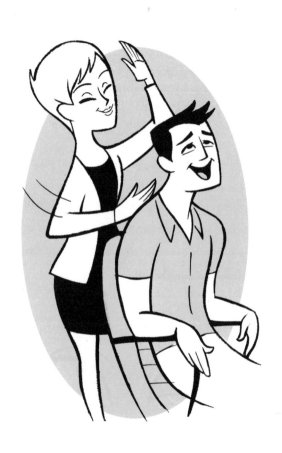

KARATE CHOP your **CUBE** *mate*

Through thick and thin, your office mates stand by your side. It's payback time!

1   Ask a workmate permission to massage him and stand behind him as he sits in his chair.

2   Do a series of gentle, short, rapid karate chops on his shoulders.

3   Work into the sore muscles along the spine.

4   Avoid bones, only do muscle!

5   Inquire about the pressure and adjust to his request.

6   Have him lean forward so you can reach the upper back on both sides of his spine.

7   Tell the recipient to close his eyes and take a breath, relaxing his shoulders.

Your workmates will be grateful for their revived muscles and refreshed minds.

 Be kind, for everyone you meet is fighting a hard battle. —Plato

BED *retreat*

The skin is the largest organ of the body. If you are sleep-deprived, your skin will show it. Make sure you get seven to nine hours of sleep, and you will wake up rosy-cheeked and refreshed.

1 Rent some relaxing videos.

2 Light a few candles, dim the lights, and turn your phone ringer off.

3 Prepare some calming chamomile or peppermint tea before bedtime.

4 Dab a drop of lavender on a tissue and place it on your pillow for a soothing scent.

MANICURE and **PEDICURE**
while you SLEEP

When you're ready for bed, prepare this miniwrap for your
hands and feet. Apply a generous amount of rich, natural
moisturizer to your hands and feet. Pull a pair of cotton
gloves or socks over your hands and put a pair of cotton
socks on your feet. When you awake, your hands and feet
will be remarkably softer.

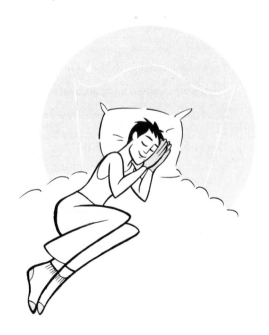

STRESS *survival KITS*

Here are some *Office Spa* kits that will help soothe and relax you all day long.

Aromatherapy Travel Kit

Create a handy aromatherapy kit for home, office, and on-the-go. You'll need a small pouch that fits the five essential oil vials:

- Eucalyptus—cool and energizing decongestant

- Ylang-ylang—uplifting and balancing, soothes mental fatigue

- Lavender—relaxing, relieves tension and aids sleep

- Peppermint—stimulating and reviving, aids digestion

- Sandalwood—warm and exotic, calming

Home Stress Survival Kit

It's nice to have supplies at home for pre- and post-work relaxation. Pamper yourself through the weekend. Don't let the spa end on Friday.

- Aromatherapy Travel Kit (above)

- Epsom salts, candles, incense

- Pumice stone and loofah scrub brushes

- Natural moisturizing cream

Desk Stress Survival Kit

Keep this kit handy for refreshment and rejuvenation. You'll need:

* A teapot and some teacups
* A selection of teas—peppermint, chamomile, ginger, ginseng, and green tea
* Sparkling water and fresh fruit
* Miso soup and other natural-soup packets
* Trail mix and power bars
* 2 small plastic bottles, one for aromatherapy spray and the other for massage oil
* A golf ball or rolling pin for feet
* Your favorite plants and flowers

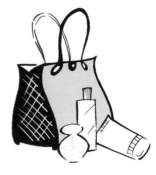

BioGRAPHIES

cole kaplan

Darrin Zeer is the author of Office Yoga and Office Spa. He has spa experience with the Four Seasons Resort, Glen Ivy Hot Springs, and the Golden Door Spa. He spent seven years in Asia traveling and studying the Eastern arts of healing.

Darrin currently lives in California and Hawaii. He spends his time writing and consulting for individuals and companies, helping them to be more calm, balanced, and effective in their work and personal lives. He is also involved in the Miracle of Love Intensive. This six-day San Francisco–based intensive attracts some eighty participants each month from around the world.

If you or your company would like to contact the author, you can visit his Web site at **www.relaxyoga.com.**

Michael Klein is an award-winning illustrator who lives just outside of New York City. His illustrations have appeared in a wide range of publications including the New York Times, Newsweek, Forbes, and Natural Health. His books include Office Yoga and The Working Stiff Cookbook, both published by Chronicle Books.

Frank Montagna is a Los Angeles–based freelance illustrator whose work has appeared in a variety of publications including New York magazine, the Wall Street Journal, Cosmo Girl, Modern Bride, and Glamour Germany. He also works in television as a production and character designer, and has done animation work for Walt Disney Feature Animation and MTV. Office Spa, published by Chronicle Books, is his first book.